THE POWER OF PLANTS

Cookbook With Over 50 Recipes to Start a
Balanced Plant-Based Alimentation

GREEN KITCHEN

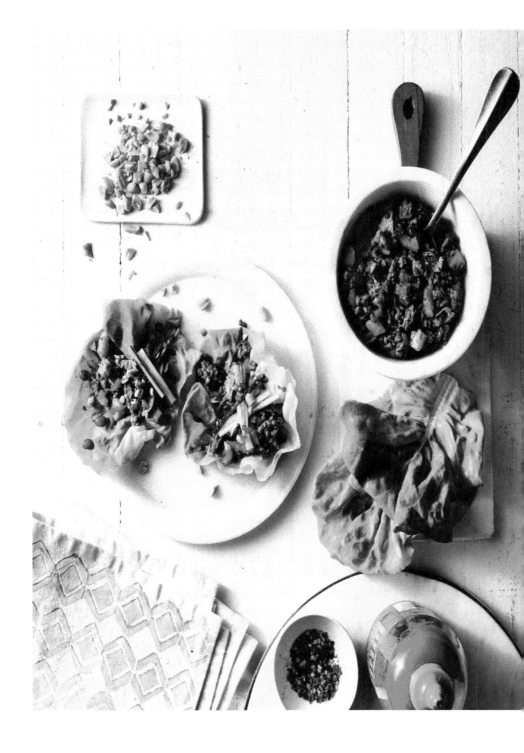

Table of Contents

INTRODUCTION

Eating healthy cannot be overemphasized, in a world where fast food and junk food is always available. We all know that we could and should be eating healthier but there are so many diets being advertised that it's hard to know what's best for you.

We're always reading about how processed foods are bad for your body. You may have also been advised repeatedly to avoid foods high in preservatives; however, no one likes to eat bland food or spend their time reading labels. This book will teach you how to find nutritious, delicious foods that will keep you satisfied while improving your health.

BENEFITS OF A BALANCED DIET

Before we dive into talking about the recipes and foods you need for a balanced diet, let's discuss a little more on the need for eating balanced diet regularly.

- IMPROVED MEMORY: I know what you are thinking. "Are you being serious right now? If I just eat a few vegetables, I can be like Einstein?" Yes! You may not be as smart as Einstein, but healthy nutrients like Vitamins D, E, and C will help improve brain functionality.

- PREVENTS CANCER: According to medical experts, eating food that contains antioxidant can help protect cells from damage, thereby leading to a reduction in the risk of getting cancer. Cancer can also be treated at its early stage with healthy food.

- EMOTIONAL STABILITY: I know what you are thinking again. "Do you mean that if I'm going through a heartbreak and I eat some healthy food, I will be better?"

  Yeah! It's not quite as straightforward as that, but healthy meals help improve your moods and balance your emotions. Scientists and researchers in 2016 found out that meals with a high glycemic load (high in carbohydrates) can trigger symptoms of depression and fatigue. Vegetables and fruits have a lower glycemic load and will help keep your blood sugar balanced.

- WEIGHT LOSS: Being overweight or obese can lead to other complicated illnesses like heart diseases, loss of bone density, and some types of cancer. Maintaining a healthful diet free from processed foods can help you stay at a healthy weight without resorting to fad diets.

- STRONG BONES AND TEETH: For healthy bones and teeth, a diet rich in calcium and magnesium is important. Maintaining bone integrity can reduce the risk of developing bone conditions later in life, such as osteoporosis.

Here are some foods are rich in calcium:

- Low-fat dairy products
- Cabbage
- Legumes
- Broccoli
- Cauliflower
- Tofu

Now you know the awesome benefits of a healthy balanced diet, I'm sure you are on the edge of your seat waiting to see the healthy and easy to make meals planned out for you. Be sure to try them out and begin eating healthier today.

Enjoy!

BREAKFAST

Classic French Toast

(Ready in 20 minutes / Servings 4).

Per servings: Calories:233; Fat: 6.5g; Carbs:35.5g; Protein: 8.2g

Ingredients

- 2 Tablespoon ground flax seeds
- 2 cup coconut Milk
- 1 teaspoon ground cinnamon
- 2 tablespoon agave syrup
- A pinch of sea salt
- A pinch of grated nutmeg
- 1 teaspoon of vanilla paste
- ½ teaspoon ground cloves

Directions

1. Meticulously Combine the coconut milk, salt, nutmeg, cinnamon, cloves, vanilla paste, agave syrup and flaxseed in a clean mixing bowl.
2. Dredge each slice of bread in the milk mixture until it is fully covered on all sides.
3. Preheat an electric griddle or a frying pan to medium heat and slightly oil it with a non-stick cooking spray. Cook each slice of bread for about 3 minutes per side on a preheated griddle until golden brown.

Enjoy.

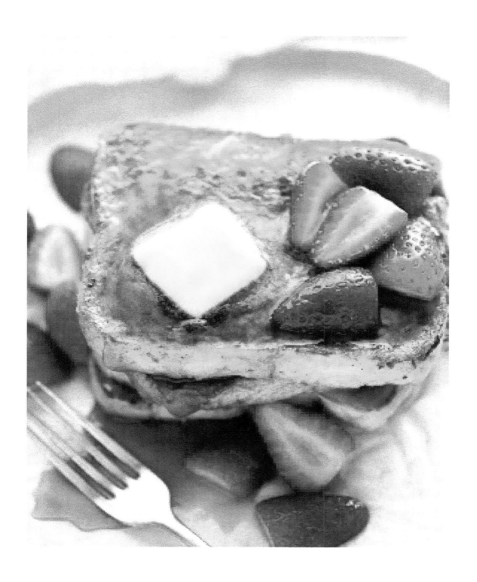

Raspberry and Chia Smoothie

(Ready in 10 minutes / servings 4)
Per serving: Calories: 442; Fat; 10.9g; Carbs; 85g;
Protein: 9.6g.

Ingredients

- 2 tablespoon coconut flakes
- 2 tablespoon pepitas
- 2 cup coconut milk
- 2 tablespoon chia seeds
- 4 small-sized bananas, peeled
- 3 cups raspberries, fresh or frozen
- 4 dates, pitted

Directions

1. Mix the coconut milk with bananas, raspberries and dates into your blender.
2. Blend until the mixture becomes smooth and creamy. Divide the smoothie into four neat bowls.
3. Place your coconut flakes, pepitas and chia seeds on each of the bowls to top it up.

Enjoy.

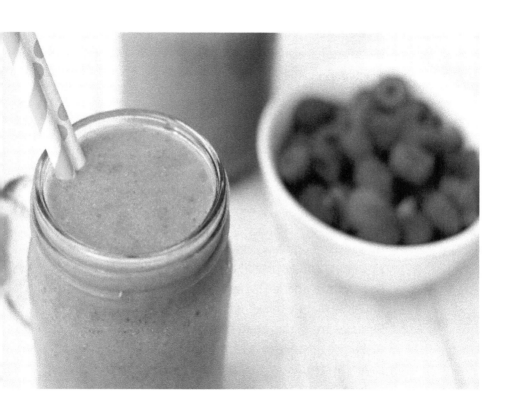

Fruit salad and Lemon- Ginger syrup

(Ready in 10 minutes/ servings 8)
Per serving; Calories:164; Fat:0.5g; Carbs: 42g; Protein; 1.4g.

Ingredients

- ½ cup agave syrup
- 2 teaspoon fresh ginger, grated
- 1 teaspoon vanilla extract
- 2 cup seedless grapes
- 4 cups apples, cored and diced
- 1 cup fresh lemon juice
- 2 bananas, sliced

Directions

1. Add the lemon juice, agave syrup, ginger to a medium-sized pot, and let it boil over medium heat. Reduce the heat a little and let it simmer for about 4 to 6 minutes until it is slightly thickened.
2. Remove from the heat and stir in the vanilla extract. Allow the mixture to cool.
3. Layer the fruits in the serving bowl. Pour the cooled sauce over the fruit and serve chilled.

Bon Appetit!

Simple Morning Polenta

(Ready in 20 minutes / servings 4)
Per serving: Calories: 306; Fat: 16g; Carbs 32.4g; Protein:7.7g.

Ingredients

- 4 Tablespoons olive oil
- 1 Tablespoon sea salt
- 1 cup cornmeal
- ½ teaspoon ground black pepper, to taste
- ½ tablespoon red pepper flakes, crushed.
- 4 cups vegetable broth

Directions

1. Boil your vegetable broth in a large saucepan over medium heat. Add in your cornmeal and keep turning it to avoid lumps
2. Season your mixture with salt, red pepper and black pepper
3. Reduce the heat so the mixture can simmer and stir periodically for about 8 to 20 minutes until the mixture is thickened.
4. Now, you can pour the olive oil into the pan, stir to combine well.

Enjoy!

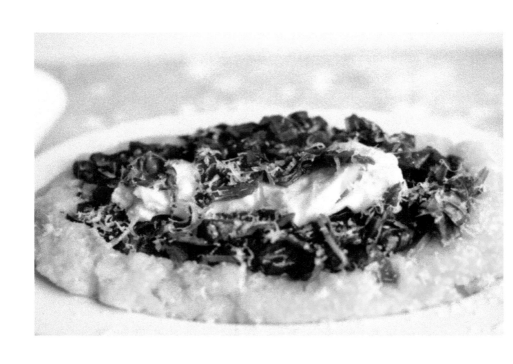

Yummy Tofu Scramble

(Ready in 15 minutes/ servings 4)
Per serving: Calories: 202; Fat:14.3; Carbs 7.5g; Protein:14.6g.

Ingredients

- 2 Tablespoon olive oil
- 12 Ounce extra firm tofu, pressed and crumbled
- 1 teaspoon garlic powder
- 1 teaspoon turmeric powder
- Sea salt and ground black pepper to taste
- ½ teaspoon cumin powder
- 2 cup baby spinach

Directions

1. Place a neat frying skillet over medium heat and heat up the olive oil. When it's hot enough, add the saute and tofu for 8 minutes, stirring periodically to promote even cooking.
2. Add into the mixture the baby spinach and aromatics and continue sauteing an additional 2 to 3 minutes
3. Garnish your mixture with fresh chives. Best served warm.

Bon Appetit!

Almond Flour English Muffins

Ready in about 20 minutes | Servings: 8

Ingredients

- 4 tbsp flax seed powder
- 1 tsp baking powder
- 2 pinches of salt
- 6 tbsp plant butter
- 4 tbsp almond flour

Directions

1. In a small bowl, mix the flaxseed with 6 tbsp water until evenly combined and leave to soak for 5 minutes. In another bowl, evenly combine the almond flour, baking powder, and salt. Then, pour in the vegan "flax egg" and whisk again. Let the batter sit for 5 minutes to set.
2. Melt plant butter in a frying pan and add the mixture in four dollops. Fry until golden brown on one side, then flip the bread with a spatula and fry further until golden brown. Serve

No-Bread Avocado Sandwich

Ready in about 10 minutes | Servings: 4

Ingredients

- 2 avocados, sliced
- 2 large red tomato, sliced
- 4 oz gem lettuce leaves
- 1 oz plant butter
- 2 oz tofu, sliced
- Freshly chopped parsley to garnish.

Directions

1. Put the avocado on a plate and place the tomato slices by the avocado. Arrange the lettuce (with the inner side facing you) on a flat plate to serve as the base of the sandwich.

2. To make the sandwich, spread plant butter on each lettuce leaf and layer tofu slices between the leaves. Then, on each cheese, place slices of avocado and tomato. Serve garnished with parsley.

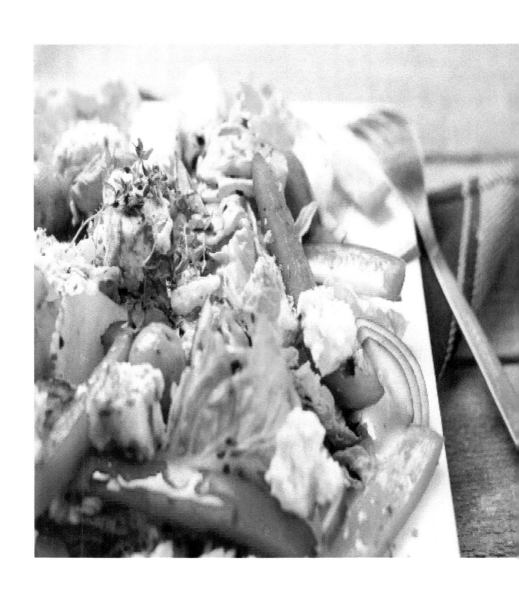

Coconut Porridge with Strawberries

Ready in about 12 minutes | Servings: 4

Ingredients

- 2 tbsp flax seed powder
- 2oz olive oil
- 2 tbsp coconut flour
- 2 pinch ground chia seeds
- 10 tbsp coconut cream
- Thawed frozen strawberries

Directions

1. Mix the flaxseed powder with the 3 tbsp water in a small bowl, and allow soaking for 5 minutes.

2. Place a non-stick saucepan over low heat and pour in the olive oil, vegan "flax egg," coconut flour, chia seeds, and coconut cream. Cook the mixture while stirring continuously until your desired consistency is achieved. Turn the heat off and spoon the porridge into serving bowls. Top with 4 to 6 strawberries and serve immediately.

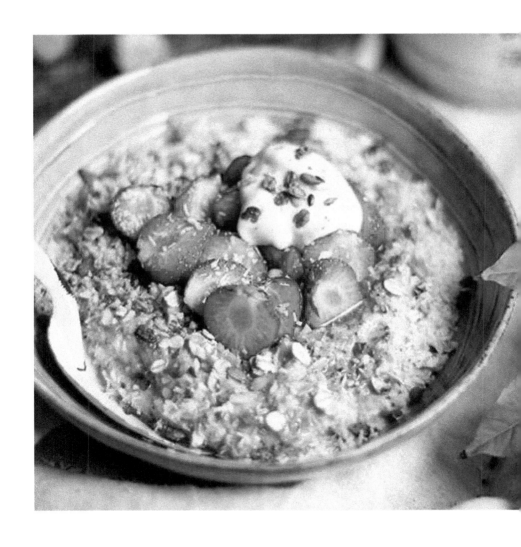

Vegan Breakfast Hash

Ready in about 25 minutes | Servings: 8
Per serving: Carbs: 29. 7g Protein: 5. 5g Fats: 10g Calories: 217 Kcal

Ingredients:

- Bell Pepper: 2
- Smoked Paprika: 1 tsp
- Potatoes: 6 medium
- Mushrooms: 16 oz
- Yellow Onion: 2
- Zucchini: 2
- Cumin Powder: 1 tsp
- Garlic Powder: 1 tsp
- Salt and Pepper: as per your taste
- Cooking oil: 4 tbsp (optional)

Directions:

1. Heat a large pan on medium flame, add oil and put the sliced potatoes
2. Cook the potatoes till they change color
3. Cut the rest of the vegetables and add all the spices
4. Cooked till veggies are soften

Vegan Muffin Sandwich

Ready in 20 minutes | Servings: 4
Per serving: Carbs: 18g Protein: 12g Fats: 14g Calories: 276 Kcal

Ingredients

- Romesco Sauce: 6-8 tablespoons
- Fresh baby spinach: 1 cup
- Tofu Scramble: 4
- Vegan English muffins: 4
- Avocado: 1 peeled and sliced
- Sliced fresh tomato: 2

Directions

1. In the oven, toast an English muffin
2. Cut Half the muffin and spread romesco sauce
3. Paste spinach to one side, tailed by avocado slices
4. Have warm tofu followed by a tomato slice
5. Place the other muffin half onto the preceding one

Enjoy!

Cauliflower and Potato Hash brown

Ready in 35 minutes | Servings: 8
Per serving: Calories 265 Fats 11. 9g Carbs 36. 7g Protein 5. 3g

Ingredients

- 6 tbsp flax seed powder + 18 tbsp water
- 4 large potatoes, peeled and shredded
- 2 big head cauliflower, rinsed and riced
- 1 white onion, grated
- 2 tsp salt
- 2 tbsp black pepper
- 8 tbsp plant butter, for frying

Directions

1. Combine the flaxseed powder and water in a medium mixing cup. Allow the flax egg to thicken for 5 minutes.
2. Toss together the potatoes, cauliflower, carrot, garlic, and black pepper with the flax egg until well mixed.
3. Allow 5 minutes for the sauce to thicken. Melt 1 tbsp plant butter in a non-stick skillet in batches, then add 4 scoops of the hash brown mixture to the skillet.
4. Make sure each scoop is separated by 1 to 2 inches. Flatten the batter with a spoon and simmer for 2 minutes, or until compacted and golden brown on the rim.
5. Cook for another 2 minutes, or until the vegetables are fried and golden brown on the other side. Transfer over a paper towel-lined plate to drain grease. Using the remaining ingredients, make the remaining hash browns.

Serve warm.

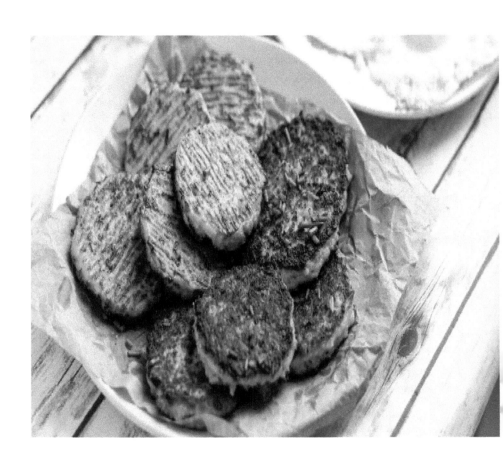

Pesto Bread Twists

Ready in about 35 minutes | Servings: 12

Ingredients

- 3 cups grated plant-based mozzarella cheese
- 8 tbsp coconut flour
- 10 tbsp plant butter
- 1 cup almond flour
- 1 tsp salt
- 2 tbsp flax seed powder
- 2 tsp baking powder
- Olive oil for brushing
- 4 oz pesto

Directions

1. First, mix the flax seed powder with 3 tbsp water in a bowl, and set aside to soak for 3 to 5 minutes.
2. Preheat oven to 350 F and line a baking sheet with parchment paper. In a bowl, evenly combine the coconut flour, almond flour, salt, and baking powder. Melt the plant butter and cheese in a deep skillet over medium heat and stir in the vegan "flax egg." Mix in the flour mixture until a firm dough forms.
3. Turn the heat off, transfer the mixture in between two parchment papers, and then use a rolling pin to flatten the dough of about an inch's thickness.
4. Remove the parchment paper on top and spread the pesto all over the dough. Now, use a knife to cut the

dough into strips, twist each piece, and place it on the baking sheet.

5. Brush with olive oil and bake for 15 to 20 minutes until golden brown.
6. Remove the bread twist; allow cooling for a few minutes, and serve with warm almond milk.

Bon Appetit!

LUNCH

Sweet Paprika Pumpkin Pasta

Preparation Time: **5 minutes** | *Cooking Time:* **10 minutes** | *Servings:* **4**

Ingredients
- 1/2 cup of coconut oil
- 1 onion
- 1 tablespoon butter
- 1 teaspoon garlic
- 1/2 teaspoon paprika
- 2 cup pumpkin purée
- 10 cups vegetable broth
- 1/2 teaspoon salt
- Freshly cracked pepper
- 2 cup pasta
- 1/4 cup coconut cream
- 1/2 cup grated mozzarella cheese

Directions
1. Add the coconut oil to the Instant Pot, hit "Sauté", Add butter and onion until it is soft and transparent. Add the garlic and paprika to the onion and sauté for about one minute more. Finally, add the pumpkin purée, vegetable broth, salt, and pepper to the Instant Pot and stir until the ingredients are combined and smooth.
2. Add pasta, then place a lid on the Instant Pot and lock it into place to seal. Pressure Cook on High Pressure for 4 minutes. Use Quick Pressure Release.
3. Add coconut cream and mozzarella cheese.

Enjoy.

Creamy Mushroom Herb Pasta

*Preparation Time: **05 minutes** | Cooking Time: **10 minutes** | Servings: **4***

Per Serving: Calories 107, Total Fat 7. 5g, Saturated Fat 4. 8g, Cholesterol 15mg, Sodium 439mg, Total Carbohydrate 5. 7g, Dietary Fiber 2. 8g, Total Sugars 1. 3g, Protein 4. 2g

Ingredients
- 1/2 cup of coconut oil
- 1 cup mushrooms
- 1 teaspoon garlic powder
- 3 tablespoon butter
- 3 tablespoon coconut flour
- 2 cup vegetable broth
- 2 sprig fresh thyme
- 1 teaspoon basil
- Salt and pepper to taste

Directions
1. Add the coconut oil to the Instant Pot, hit "Sauté", add butter, when the butter melts, add garlic powder, add the sliced mushrooms and continue to cook until the mushrooms have turned dark brown and all of the moisture they release has evaporated.
2. Add the flour, Whisk the vegetable broth into the Instant Pot with the flour and mushrooms. Add the thyme, basil, and some freshly cracked pepper.

3. Then add pasta, place the lid on the pot and lock it into place to seal. Pressure Cook on High Pressure for 4 minutes. Use Quick Pressure Release.

Serve and enjoy.

Enjoy!

Lemon Garlic Broccoli Macaroni

Preparation Time: 5 minutes | Cooking Time: 10 minutes | Servings: 4

Per Serving: Calories 254, Total Fat 7. 4g, Saturated Fat 3. 9g, Cholesterol 62mg, Sodium 66mg, Total Carbohydrate 39. 8g, Dietary Fibre 1. 5g, Total Sugars 1. 3g, Protein 8. 4g

Ingredients

- 2 cup macaroni
- 1 cup broccoli
- 1 tablespoon butter
- 1 teaspoon garlic powder
- 2 lemon
- Salt and pepper to taste
- Enough water

Directions

1. Add macaroni, butter, water, broccoli, lemon, garlic powder, and salt to Instant Pot.
2. Place the lid on the pot and lock it into place to seal. Pressure Cook on High Pressure for 4 minutes. Use Quick Pressure Release.

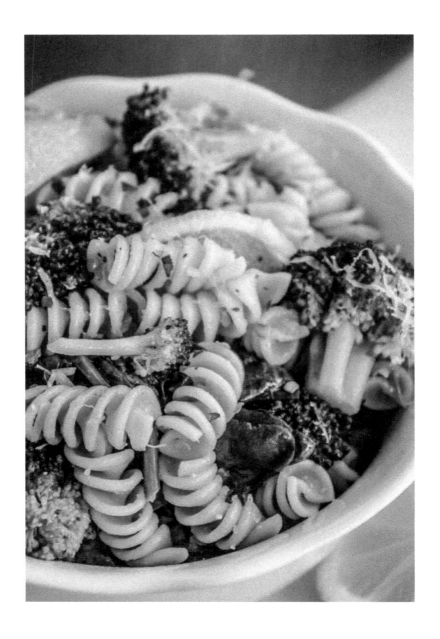

Tasty Pasta Eggplant Sauce

Preparation Time: **05 minutes** | *Cooking Time:* **10 minutes** | *Servings:* **2**

Per Serving: Calories 306, Total Fat 18g, Saturated Fat 12. 9g, Cholesterol 30mg, Sodium 188mg, Total Carbohydrate 27g, Dietary Fibre 12. 6g 45%, Total Sugars 13. 9g, Protein 14. 2g

Ingredients

- 2 tablespoon coconut oil
- 4 cloves garlic
- 2 small onion
- 2 medium eggplant
- 2 cup diced tomatoes
- 2 tablespoon tomato sauce
- 1/2 teaspoon dried thyme
- 1 teaspoon honey
- Pinch paprika
- Freshly cracked pepper
- 1/2 salt and pepper, or to taste
- 12 oz. spaghetti
- 4 cups vegetable broth
- Handful fresh coriander, chopped

Directions

1. Set Instant Pot to Sauté. Add the coconut oil and allow it to melt. Add the onion and garlic and cook for 2 minutes or until the onion is soft and transparent.

2. Add eggplant, diced tomatoes, tomato sauce, thyme, honey, paprika, and freshly cracked pepper. Stir them well to combine, Add spaghetti, and vegetable broth, salt, and pepper.
3. Lock the lid and make sure the vent is closed. Set Instant Pot to Manual or Pressure Cook on High Pressure for 10 minutes. When cooking time ends, release pressure and wait for steam to completely stop before opening the lid.
4. Top each serving with grated goat and a sprinkle of fresh coriander.

Tasty Mac and Cheese

*Preparation Time:**05 minutes** | Cooking Time: **15 minutes** | Servings: **4***

Per Serving: Calories 210, Total Fat 3g, Saturated Fat 1g, Cholesterol 4mg, Sodium 374mg, Total Carbohydrate 35. 7g, Dietary Fibre 1. 8g, Total Sugars 3. 6g, Protein 9. 6g

Ingredients
- 1 cup of soy milk
- 2 cup dry macaroni
- Enough water
- 1/2 teaspoon salt
- 1 cup shredded mozzarella cheese
- 1/2 teaspoon Dijon mustard
- 1/4 teaspoon red chili powder

Directions
1. Add macaroni, soy milk, water, and salt, chili powder, Dijon mustard to the Instant Pot or pressure cooker. Place lid on Instant Pot and lock into place to seal.
2. Pressure Cook on High Pressure for 4 minutes. Use Quick Pressure Release. Stir cheese into macaroni and then stir in the cheeses until well melted and combined.

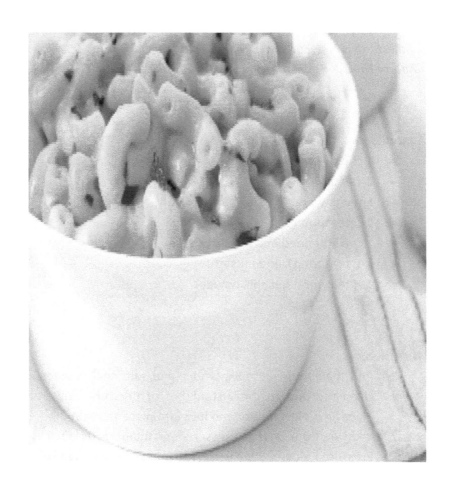

Simple Spinach Ricotta Pasta

*Preparation Time:**05 minutes** | Cooking Time:**20 minutes** | Servings: **4***

Per Serving: Calories 277, Total Fat 18.9g, Saturated Fat 15.2g, Cholesterol 16mg, Sodium 191mg, Total Carbohydrate 23.8g, Dietary Fiber 1.2g, Total Sugars 1.4g, Protein 5.1g

Ingredients

- 1 cup pasta
- 2 cup vegetable broth
- 1 lb. uncooked tagliatelle
- 2 tablespoon coconut oil
- 1 teaspoon garlic powder
- 1/2 cup almond milk
- 1 cup whole milk ricotta
- 1/4 teaspoon salt
- Freshly cracked pepper
- 1/2 cup chopped spinach

Directions

1. Add the vegetable broth, tagliatelle, spinach, salt, some freshly cracked pepper, and the pasta. Place lid on Instant Pot and lock into place to seal.
2. Pressure Cook on High Pressure for 4 minutes. Use Quick Pressure Release.
3. Prepare the ricotta sauce. Mince the garlic and add it to a large skillet with coconut oil. Cook over Medium-Low

heat for 2-3 minutes, or just until soft and fragrant (but not browned). Add the almond milk and ricotta, then stir until relatively smooth (the ricotta may be slightly grainy).

4. Allow the sauce to heat through and come to a low simmer. The sauce will thicken slightly as it simmers. Once it's thick enough to coat the spoon (4-6 minutes), season with salt and pepper.

5. Add the cooked and drained pasta to the sauce and toss to coat. If the sauce becomes too thick or dry, add a small amount of the reserved pasta cooking water. Serve warm.

Enjoy!

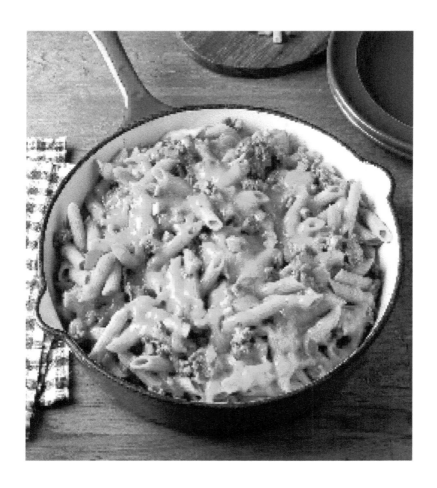

Basil Spaghetti Pasta

Preparation Time: **5 minutes** | *Cooking Time:* **10 minutes** | *Servings:* **4**

Per Serving: Calories 216, Total Fat 2.3g, Saturated Fat 0.7g, Cholesterol 49mg, Sodium 160mg, Total Carbohydrate 36g, Dietary Fiber 0.1g, Total Sugars 0.4g, Protein 12.2g

Ingredients
- 1 teaspoon garlic powder
- 2 cup spaghetti
- 4 large eggs
- 1/2 cup grated Parmesan cheese
- Freshly cracked pepper
- Salt and pepper to taste
- Handful fresh basil
- Enough water

Directions
1. In a medium bowl, whisk together the eggs, 1/2 cup of the Parmesan cheese, and a generous dose of freshly cracked pepper.
2. Add spaghetti, water, basil, garlic powder, pepper, and salt to Instant Pot. Place lid on Instant Pot and lock into place to seal. Pressure Cook on High Pressure for 4 minutes. Use Quick Pressure Release.
3. Pour the eggs and Parmesan mixture over the hot pasta.

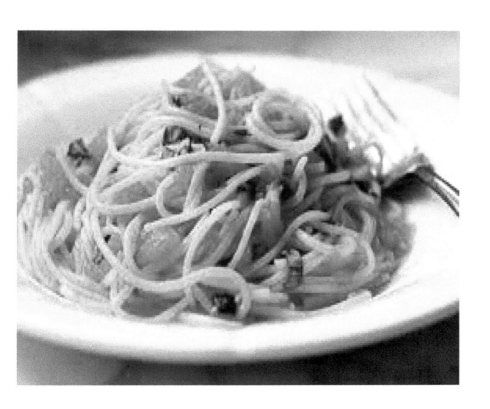

Cabbage and Noodles

*Preparation Time: **15 minutes** | Cooking Time: **10 minutes** | Servings: **4***

Per Serving: Calories 183, Total Fat 6.8g, Saturated Fat 3.9g, Cholesterol 31mg, Sodium 78mg, Total Carbohydrate 27.2g, Dietary Fibre 5.9g, Total Sugars 7.6g, Protein 5.4g

Ingredients

- 2 cup wide egg noodles
- 3 tablespoon butter
- 2 small onion
- 1 head green cabbage, shredded
- Salt and pepper to taste

Directions

1. Add egg noodles, butter, water, onion, green cabbage, pepper, and salt to Instant Pot. Place lid on Instant Pot and lock into place to seal.
2. Pressure Cook on High Pressure for 4 minutes. Use Quick Pressure Release.

Serve and enjoy.

Tasty Penne with Vegetables

Preparation Time: 5 minutes | Cooking Time: 10 minutes | Servings: 4

Per Serving: Calories 381, Total Fat 13. 2g, Saturated Fat 8. 7g, Cholesterol 56mg, Sodium 1006mg, Total Carbohydrate 52. 3g, Dietary Fibre 4. 7g, Total Sugars 8. 6g, Protein 15. 3g

Ingredients
- 1 tablespoon butter
- 2 cup penne
- 2 small onion
- 1 teaspoon garlic powder
- 2 carrot
- 1 red bell pepper
- 1 pumpkin
- 4 cups vegetable broth
- 4 oz. coconut cream
- 1/4 cup grated Parmesan cheese
- 1/4 teaspoon salt and pepper to taste
- Dash hot sauce, optional
- ½ cup cauliflower florets

Directions
1. Set Instant Pot to Sauté. Add the butter and allow it to melt. Add the onion and garlic powder and cook for 2 minutes. Stir regularly.

2. Add the carrot, red pepper and pumpkin, and cauliflower to the pot.
3. Add penne, vegetable broth, coconut cream, salt, and pepper then add hot sauce.
4. Lock the lid and make sure the vent is closed. Set Instant Pot to Manual or Pressure Cook on High Pressure for 10 minutes. When cooking time ends, release pressure and wait for steam to stop before opening the lid completely.
5. Stir in cheese, sprinkle a bit on top of the pasta when you serve it.

Pasta with Eggplant Sauce

Preparation Time: **5 minutes** | *Cooking Time:* **10 minutes** | *Servings:* **4**

Per Serving: Calories 306, Total Fat 18g, Saturated Fat 12.9g, Cholesterol 30mg, Sodium 188mg, Total Carbohydrate 27g, Dietary Fibre 12.6g 45%, Total Sugars 13.9g, Protein 14.2g

Ingredients
- 2 tablespoon coconut oil
- 4 cloves garlic
- 2 small onion
- 2 mediums eggplant
- 2 cup diced tomatoes
- 2 tablespoon tomato sauce
- 1/2 teaspoon dried thyme
- 1 teaspoon honey
- Pinch paprika
- Freshly cracked pepper
- 1/2 salt and pepper, or to taste
- 12 oz. spaghetti
- 4 cups vegetable broth
- Handful fresh coriander, chopped

Directions

1. Set Instant Pot to Sauté. Add the coconut oil and allow it to melt. Add the onion and garlic and cook for 2 minutes or until the onion is soft and transparent.
2. Add eggplant, diced tomatoes, tomato sauce, thyme, honey, paprika, and freshly cracked pepper. Stir them well to combine, Add spaghetti, and vegetable broth, salt, and pepper.
3. Lock the lid and make sure the vent is closed. Set Instant Pot to Manual or Pressure Cook on High Pressure for 10 minutes. When cooking time ends, release pressure and wait for steam to stop before opening the lid completely.
4. Top each with sprinkle of fresh coriander.

Enjoy!

Sweet Peanut Noodles Stir Fry

Preparation Time: 5 minutes | Cooking Time: 17 minutes | Servings: 4

Per Serving: Calories 501, Total Fat 24. 4g, Saturated Fat 4. 6g, Cholesterol 1mg, Sodium 788mg, Total Carbohydrate 58. 1g, Dietary Fiber 6g, Total Sugars 15. 8g, Protein 17. 3g

Ingredients
- 1 teaspoon ginger powder
- ½ cup natural peanut butter
- 1/2 cup hoisin sauce
- 2 cup hot water
- ½ teaspoon sriracha hot sauce
- 2 tablespoon vegetable oil
- 1 teaspoon garlic powder
- 2 cup frozen stir fry vegetables
- 4 oz. soba noodles
- 4 sliced leeks, optional

Directions
1. Prepare the sauce first. Add ginger powder into a bowl. Add the peanut butter, hoisin sauce, sriracha hot sauce, and ¼ cup of hot water. Stir or whisk until smooth. Set the sauce aside until it is needed.
2. Set the Instant Pot to Sauté. Add the vegetable oil and allow it to sizzle. Add garlic powder and ginger powder

and cook for 2 minutes. Add the bag of frozen vegetables and cook for 5 minutes. Add the remaining water and soba noodles.

3. Lock the lid and make sure the vent is closed. Set Instant Pot to Manual or Pressure Cook on High Pressure for 10 minutes. When cooking time ends, release pressure and wait for steam to stop before opening the lid completely.

4. Stir until everything is combined and coated with sauce. Garnish with sliced leek if desired.

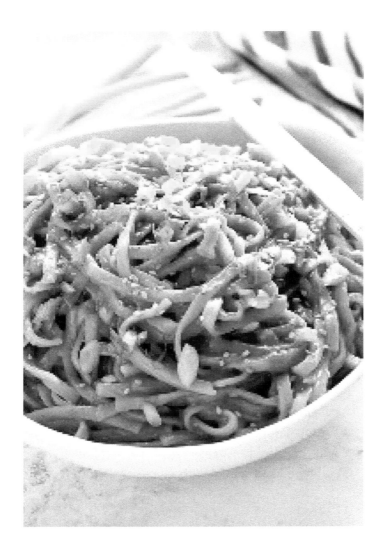

Lemon Mozzarella Pasta

Preparation Time: 5 minutes | Cooking Time: 10 minutes | Servings: 4

Per Serving: Calories 273, Total Fat 5. 9g, Saturated Fat 1. 3g, Cholesterol 4mg, Sodium 44mg, Total Carbohydrate 46. 6g, Dietary Fibre 3. 7g, Total Sugars 2. 8g, Protein 10. 3g.

Ingredients:
- 8 oz. macaroni
- ½ cup peas
- 1 cup mozzarella cheese
- 1 tablespoon olive oil
- 2 lemon
- Salt and pepper

Directions:
- Set Instant Pot to Sauté. Add the olive oil and allow it to sizzle. Add macaroni, peas, lemon, salt, and pepper.
- Lock the lid and make sure the vent is closed. Set Pot to Pressure Cook on High Pressure for 10 minutes. When cooking time ends, release pressure and wait for steam to stop before opening the lid completely.
- Add mozzarella cheese and Stir until everything is combined and coated with sauce.

Enjoy.

Creamy Soup of Zucchini with Walnuts

Preparation Time: 45 minutes | *Servings:* 4

Ingredients

- 3 zucchinis, chopped
- 2 tsp olive oil
- Sea salt and black pepper to taste
- 1 onion, diced
- 4 cups vegetable stock
- 3 tsp ground sage
- 3 tbsp nutritional yeast
- 1 cup non-dairy milk
- ¼ cup toasted walnuts

Directions

1. Heat the oil in a skillet and place zucchini, onion, salt, and pepper; cook for 5 minutes. Pour in vegetable stock and bring to a boil. Lower the heat and simmer for 15 minutes.
2. Stir in sage, nutritional yeast, and milk. Purée the soup with a blender until smooth. Serve garnished with toasted walnuts and pepper.

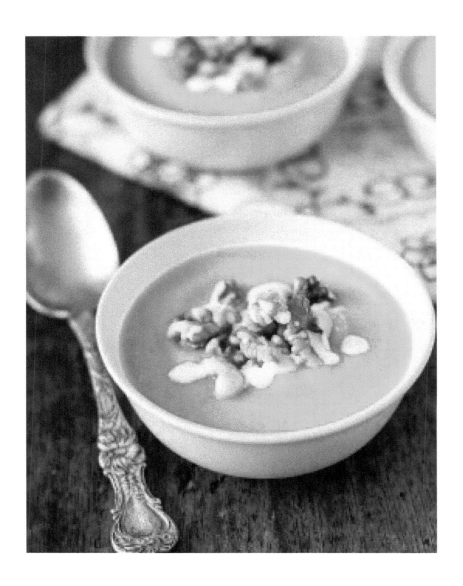

Homemade Ramen Soup

Preparation Time: 25 minutes | Servings: 4

Ingredients

- 7 oz Japanese buckwheat noodles
- 4 tbsp sesame paste
- 1 cup canned pinto beans, drained
- 2 tbsp fresh cilantro, chopped
- 2 scallions, thinly sliced

Directions

1. In boiling salted water, add in the noodles and cook for 5 minutes over low heat.
2. Remove a cup of the noodle water to a bowl and add in the sesame paste; stir until it has dissolved.
3. Pour the sesame mix in the pot with the noodles, add in pinto beans, and stir until everything is hot. Serve topped with cilantro and scallions in individual bowls.

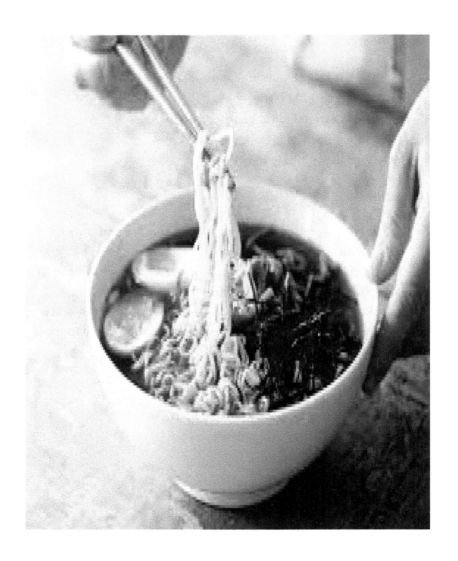

Cauliflower Soup with Leeks

Preparation Time: 25 minutes | *Servings:* 4

Ingredients

- 2 tbsp olive oil
- 3 leeks, thinly sliced
- 1 head cauliflower, cut into florets
- 4 cups vegetable stock
- Salt and black pepper to taste
- 3 tbsp chopped fresh chives

Directions

1. Heat the oil in a pot over medium heat. Place the leeks and sauté for 5 minutes.
2. Add in broccoli, vegetable stock, salt, and pepper and cook for 10 minutes.
3. Blend the soup until purée in a food processor. Top with chives and serve.

Enjoy!

Rice Noodle Soup with Beans

Preparation Time: *10 minutes* | **Servings:** *6*

Ingredients

- 2 carrots, chopped
- 2 celery stalks, chopped
- 6 cups vegetable broth
- 8 oz brown rice noodles
- 1 (15-oz) can pinto beans
- 1 tsp dried herbs

Directions

1. Place a pot over medium heat and add in the carrots, celery, and vegetable broth.
2. Bring to a boil. Add in noodles, beans, dried herbs, salt, and pepper.
3. Reduce the heat and simmer for 5 minutes. Serve.

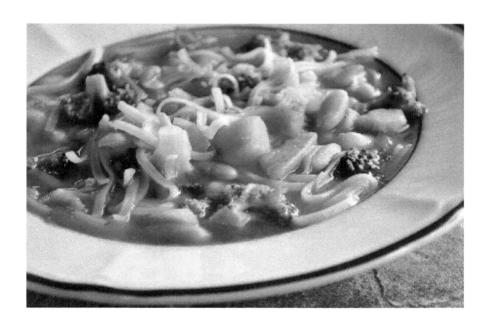

DINNER

Avocado Broccoli soup

Preparation Time: **25 minutes** | *Cooking Time:* **15-60 minutes** |
Servings: **8**

Per Serving: Calories 269; Fat 21.5 g; Carbohydrates 12.8 g; Sugar 2.1 g; Protein 9.2 g; Cholesterol 0 mg

Ingredients:
- 4 cups broccoli florets, chopped
- 10 cups vegetable broth
- 4 avocados, chopped
- Pepper
- Salt

Directions:
1. Cook broccoli in boiling water for 5 minutes. Drain well.
2. Add broccoli, vegetable broth, avocados, pepper, and salt to the blender and blend until smooth.
3. Stir well and serve warm.

Enjoy!!

African Pineapple Peanut stew

Preparation Time: 30 mins. | Cooking Time: 15-60 minutes | Servings: 8

Per Serving: 382 Calories, 20.3 g Total Fat, 0 mg Cholesterol, 27.6 g Total Carbohydrates, 5 g Dietary Fiber, 11.4 g Protein.

Ingredients
- 8 cups sliced kale
- 2 cup chopped onion
- 1 cup peanut butter
- 2 tbsp. hot pepper sauce or 1 tbsp. Tabasco sauce
- 4 minced garlic cloves
- 1 cup chopped cilantro
- 4 cups pineapple, undrained, canned & crushed
- 2 tbsp. vegetable oil

Directions
1. In a saucepan (preferably covered), sauté the garlic and onions in the oil until the onions are lightly browned, approximately 10 minutes, stirring often.
2. Wash the kale. Get rid of the stems. Mound the leaves on a cutting surface & slice crosswise into slices.
3. Now put the pineapple and juice to the onions & bring to a simmer. Stir the kale in, cover, and simmer until just tender, stirring periodically for approximately 5 minutes.
4. Mix in the hot pepper sauce, peanut butter & simmer for another 5 minutes.
5. Add salt according to your taste.

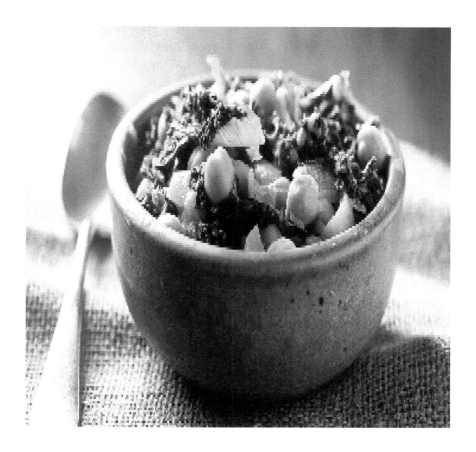

Split pea and carrot stew

Preparation Time: 10 minutes | Cooking Time: 20 minutes | Servings: 8

Per Serving: Calories 337, Total Fat 20. 5g, Saturated Fat 4. 2g, Cholesterol 0mg, Sodium 661mg, Total Carbohydrate 32. 6g, Dietary Fiber 16. 3g, Total Sugars 7. 9g, Protein 10g

Ingredients
- 2 tablespoon avocado oil
- 2 small onion, diced
- 1 carrot, diced into small cubes
- 1 leek stick, diced into cubes
- 4–5 cloves garlic, diced finely
- 2 bay leaf
- 2 teaspoon paprika powder
- 1 teaspoon cumin powder
- 1 teaspoon salt
- 1/2 teaspoon cinnamon powder
- 1/2 teaspoon chili powder or cayenne pepper
- 4 cups green split peas (rinsed well
- ½ cup chopped tinned tomatoes
- Juice of ½ lemon
- 2 cups vegetable stock

Directions

- Press the Sauté key to the Instant Pot. Add the avocado oil, onions, carrots, and leeks and cook for 4 minutes, stirring a few times.
- Add the rest of the ingredients and stir. Cancel the Sauté function by pressing the Keep Warm/Cancel button.
- Place and lock the lid, make sure the steam releasing handle is pointing to Sealing. Press Manual and adjust to 10 minutes.
- Once the timer goes off, allow the pressure to release for 4-5 minutes and then use the Quick-release method before opening the lid.

Serve.

Enjoy!

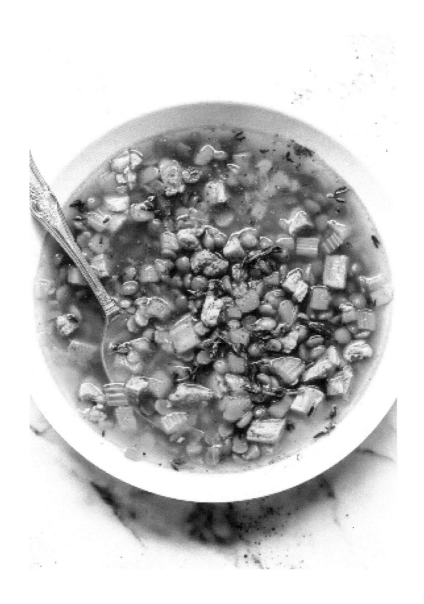

Fuss Free Cabbage tomato stew

Preparation Time: 15-30 minutes | *Cooking Time:* 3 hours and 10 minutes | *Servings:* 12

Ingredients
- 2 medium-sized cabbage head, chopped
- 2 medium-sized white onion, peeled and sliced
- 56-ounce of stewed tomatoes
- 3/2 teaspoon of salt
- 1/2 teaspoon of ground black pepper
- 20-ounce of tomato soup

Directions
1. Using a 6 quarts slow cooker, place all the ingredients, and stir properly.
2. Cover it with the lid, plug in the slow cooker and let it cook at the high heat setting for 3 hours or until the vegetables get soft.
3. Serve right away.

Creamy Garlic Onion Soup

Preparation Time: 45 minutes | Cooking Time: 15-60 minutes | Servings: 8

Per Serving: Calories 90; Fat 7.4 g; Carbohydrates 10.1 g; Sugar 4.1 g; Protein 1 g; Cholesterol 0 mg

Ingredients
- 2 onion, sliced
- 8 cups vegetable stock
- 1 tbsp olive oil
- 2 shallot, sliced
- 4 garlic clove, chopped
- 2 leek, sliced
- Salt

Directions
1. Add stock and olive oil in a saucepan and bring to boil.
2. Add remaining ingredients and stir well.
3. Cover and simmer for 25 minutes.
4. Puree the soup using an immersion blender until smooth.
5. Stir well and serve warm.

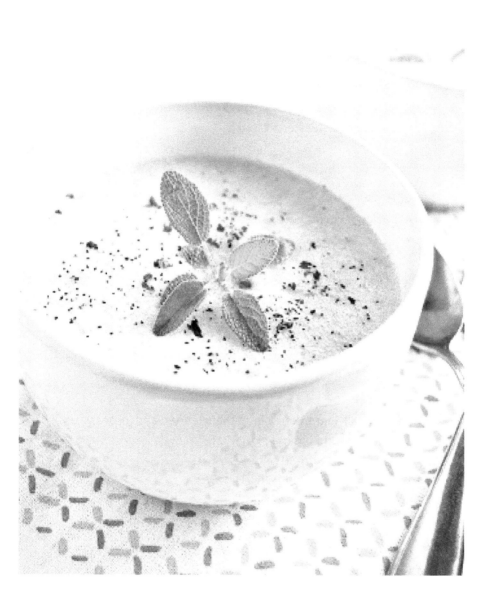

Healthy Avocado Cucumber soup

Preparation Time: 40 minutes | Cooking Time: 15-60 minutes | Servings: 6

Per Serving: Calories 73; Fat 3.7 g; Carbohydrates 9.2 g; Sugar 2.8 g; Protein 2.2 g; Cholesterol 0 mg

Ingredients:
- 2 large cucumber, peeled and sliced
- 3/2 cup of water
- 1/2 cup lemon juice
- 4 garlic cloves
- 12 green onion
- 4 avocados, pitted
- 1 tsp black pepper
- 1 tsp pink salt

Directions:
1. Add all ingredients into the blender and process until smooth and creamy.
2. Refrigerate for 30 minutes
3. Stir well and serve chilled.

Enjoy!

Tasty Zucchini soup

Preparation Time: 20 minutes | Cooking Time: 15-60 minutes | Servings: 16

Per Serving: Calories 62; Fat 4 g; Carbohydrates 6.8 g; Sugar 3.3 g; Protein 2 g; Cholesterol 0 mg

Ingredients
- 5 lbs zucchini, peeled and sliced
- 2/3 cup basil leaves
- 8 cups vegetable stock
- 8 garlic cloves, chopped
- 4 tbsp olive oil
- 2 medium onion, diced
- Pepper
- Salt

Directions
1. Heat olive oil in a pan over medium-low heat.
2. Add zucchini and onion and sauté until softened. Add garlic and sauté for a minute.
3. Add vegetable stock and simmer for 15 minutes.
4. Remove from heat. Stir in basil and puree the soup using a blender until smooth and creamy. Season with pepper and salt.
5. Stir well and serve.

Enjoy!

Vegetables in Tomatoes

Preparation Time: 5 minutes | **Cooking Time:** 24 minutes | **Servings:** 8

Ingredients
- 2 tablespoon olive oil
- 4 cloves of garlic
- 2 large onion, chopped
- 2 cup diced carrots
- 1 cup peas
- 64 ounces vegetable broth
- 2 cup broccoli florets
- 2 14-ounce can diced tomatoes
- 4 tablespoons fresh basil
- 6 cups of water
- salt and pepper to taste

Directions
1. Press the Sauté button on the Instant Pot and heat the oil. Sauté the garlic and onion until fragrant for 30 seconds or until fragrant.
2. Stir in the carrots and peas and stir for 2 minutes.
3. Add in the rest of the ingredients. Give a good stir.
4. Close the lid and set the vent to the Sealing position.
5. Press the Broth/Soup button and cook on high. Adjust the cooking time to 20 minutes.
6. Do natural pressure release.

Enjoy!

Vegetarian Mushroom Soup

Preparation Time: 5 minutes | **Cooking Time:** 6 minutes | **Servings:** 8

Ingredients

- 16 ounces sliced cremini mushrooms
- 2 cup frozen peas
- 2 onion, chopped
- 2 14-ounce diced tomatoes
- 1 cup of water
- 1 teaspoon ground cumin
- 3 cup of coconut milk
- 2 tablespoon grated ginger
- salt to taste
- 2 tablespoon sugar
- 1 cup cilantro, chopped

Directions

1. In the Instant Pot, combine the mushrooms, peas, onions, tomatoes, water, cumin, coconut milk, and ginger. Season with salt, and sugar.
2. Close the lid and set the vent to the Sealing position. Press the Pressure Cook or Manual button and adjust the cooking time to 6 minutes.
3. Do natural pressure release.
4. Once the lid is open, stir in the cilantro before serving.

Enjoy!

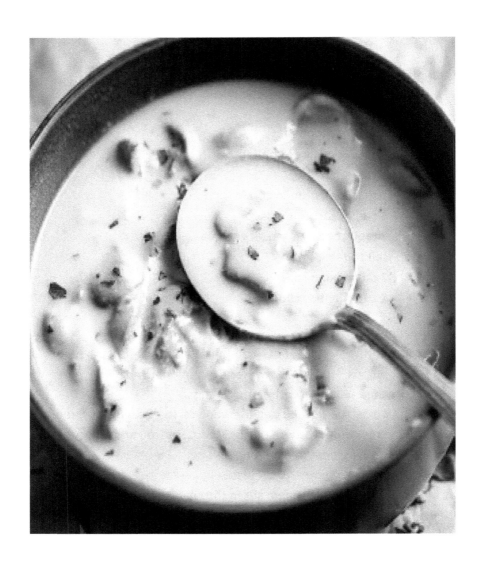

Steamed Asian Brussels Sprouts

Preparation Time: 10 minutes | Cooking Time: 20 minutes | Servings: 8

Per Serving: Calories 137, Total Fat 11g, Saturated Fat 2g, Total Carbs 8g, Net Carbs 6g, Protein 4g, Sugar: 3g, Fiber: 2g, Sodium: 137mg, Potassium: 205mg, Phosphorus: 63mg.

Ingredients

- 2 cups of water
- 4 tablespoons sesame oil
- 8 teaspoons soy sauce
- 4 teaspoon rice vinegar
- 3 cups Brussels sprouts, thinly sliced
- salt to taste
- 4 tablespoons chopped peanuts, toasted

Directions

1. Pour water into the Instant Pot and place a steamer basket or trivet inside.
2. In a heat-proof dish, mix all ingredients except for the peanuts. Toss to coat the Brussels sprouts with the ingredients.
3. Place the dish with the Brussels sprouts on the trivet.
4. Close the lid and set the vent to the Sealing position.
5. Press the Steam button and cook for 10 minutes.
6. Do natural pressure release to open the lid.
7. Garnish with toasted peanuts before serving.

Enjoy!

Smoky Veggie Chili

Preparation Time: 5 minutes | Cooking Time: 37 minutes | Servings: 10

Per Serving: Calories 586, Total Fat 4g, Saturated Fat 0.7g, Total Carbs 126g, Net Carbs 108g, Protein 15g, Sugar: 14g, Fiber: 18g, Sodium: 123mg, Potassium: 3131mg, Phosphorus: 426mg

Ingredients

- 2 tablespoon olive oil
- 4 onions, chopped
- 2 teaspoon cumin seeds
- 4 teaspoons smoked paprika
- 4 teaspoons cocoa powder
- 2 tablespoon peanut butter
- 2 fresh chilies, chopped
- 6 mixed color peppers, seeded and chopped
- 6 large tomatoes, chopped
- 4 sweet potatoes, peeled and cubed
- 16 small jacket potatoes
- 2 bunch fresh coriander, chopped
- salt and pepper to taste
- 2 cups of water

Directions

1. Press the Sauté button on the Instant Pot and heat the oil.
2. Sauté the onions and cumin until fragrant.

3. Stir in the paprika, cocoa powder, peanut butter, chili, peppers, tomatoes, and potatoes.
4. Season with salt and pepper and pour in water.
5. Close the lid and set the vent to the Sealing position.
6. Press the Meat/Stew button and cook using the present cooking time.
7. Do natural pressure release.

Enjoy!

Instant Pot Ratatouille

Preparation Time: 10 minutes | Cooking Time: 20 minutes | Servings: 8

Per Serving: Calories 354, Total Fat 7g, Saturated Fat 0.8g, Total Carbs 58g, Net Carbs 45g, Protein 15g, Sugar: 13g, Fibre: 13g, Sodium: 558mg, Potassium: 891mg, Phosphorus: 321mg.

Ingredients

- 3 tablespoon extra-virgin olive oil
- 2 tablespoon minced garlic
- 2 cup chopped red onion
- 2 cup chopped red bell pepper
- 3 14-ounce cans diced tomatoes
- 2 large zucchinis, sliced into 1inch pieces
- 2 large yellow squash, sliced into 1-inch pieces
- 2 small eggplant, peeled and slice into 1-inch pieces
- 2 tablespoon red wine vinegar
- 1 teaspoon smoked paprika
- salt to taste
- 4 tablespoons fresh basil leaves

Directions:

1. Press the Sauté button on the Instant Pot and heat the oil. Sauté the garlic, onion, and bell pepper until fragrant.
2. Stir in the tomatoes and cook for another 3 minutes.
3. Add in the zucchini, yellow squash, and eggplant.
4. Season with red wine vinegar, paprika, and salt. Top with basil.

5. Close the lid and set the vent to the Sealing position.
6. Press the Pressure Cook or Manual button and adjust the cooking time to 5 minutes.
7. Do natural pressure release.

ENJOY!

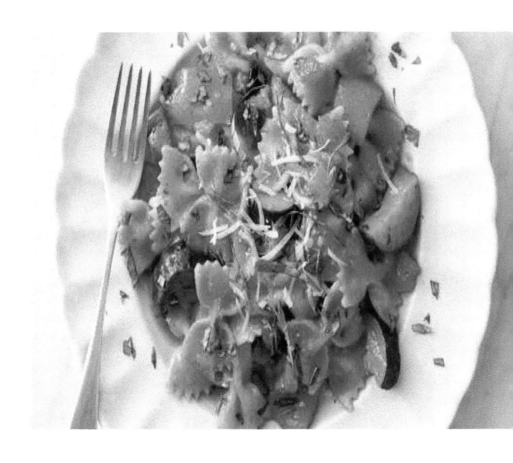

Spicy Steamed Broccoli

(Ready in 15 minutes / servings 12)

Ingredients

- 2 large head broccoli, into florets
- Salt to taste
- 2 tsp red pepper flakes

Directions

1. Boil 1 cup water in a pot over medium heat. Place in a steamer basket and put in the florets. Steam covered for 5-7 minutes.
2. In a bowl, toss the broccoli with red pepper flakes and salt. Serve.

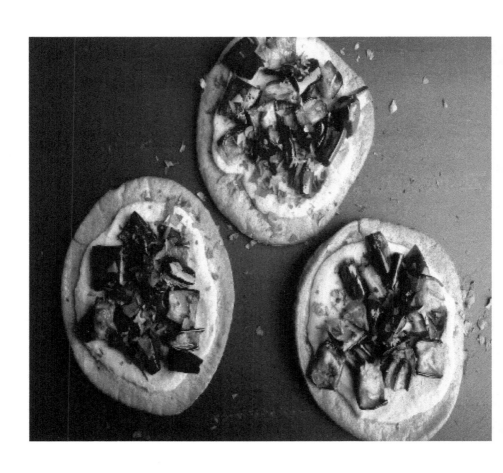

Eggplant and Humunus Pizza

(Ready in 25 minutes / servings 4)

Ingredients

- 1 eggplant, sliced
- 1 red onion, sliced
- 2 cup cherry tomatoes, halved
- 6 tbsp chopped black olives
- Salt to taste
- Drizzle olive oil
- 4 prebaked pizza crusts
- 1 cup hummus
- 4 tbsp oregano

Directions

1. Preheat oven to 390 F,
2. In a bowl, combine the eggplant, onion, tomatoes, olives, and salt. Toss to coat. Sprinkle with some olive oil.
3. Arrange the crusts on a baking sheet and spread the hummus on each pizza.
4. Top with the eggplant mixture. Bake for 20-30 minutes. Serve warm.

Miso Green Cabbage

(Ready in 50 minutes / servings 8)

Ingredients

- 2 lb. green cabbage, halved
- 4 tsp olive
- 6 tsp miso paste
- 2 tsp dried oregano
- 1 tsp dried rosemary
- 2 tbsp balsamic vinegar

Directions

1. Preheat oven to 390 F. Line with parchment paper a baking sheet.
2. Put the green cabbage in a bowl. Coat with olive oil, miso, oregano, rosemary, salt, and pepper. Remove to the baking sheet and bake for 35-40 minutes, shaking every 5 minutes until tender. Remove from the oven to a plate. Drizzle with balsamic vinegar and serve.

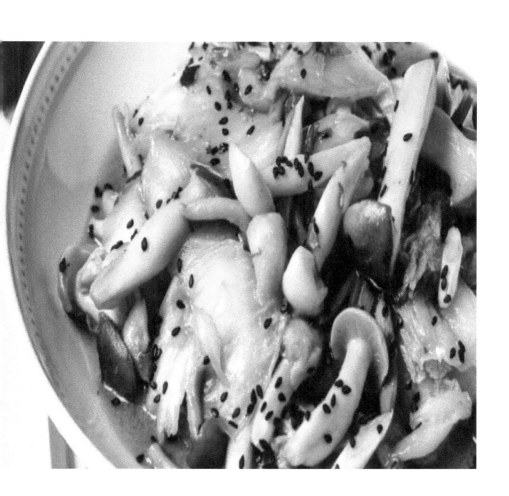

Cilantro Okra

(Ready in 10 minutes / servings 8)

Ingredients

- 4 tbsp. olive oil
- 8 cups okra, halved
- Sea salt and black pepper to taste
- 6 tbsp chopped fresh cilantro

Directions

1. Heat the oil in a skillet over medium heat. Place in the okra, cook for 5 minutes.
2. Turn the heat off and mix in salt, pepper, and cilantro. Serve immediately.

Bon Appetit!

DESSERT

Berry Compote Pancake

Ready in 30 minutes| Servings: 4

Per serving: Carbs 92g: Protein 9.4g: Fats 5.2g: Calories 463 Kcal

Ingredients

- Mixed frozen berries: 200g
- Plain flour: 140 g
- Unsweetened almond milk: 140ml
- Icing sugar: 2 tbsp
- Lemon juice: 2 tbsp
- Baking powder: 4 tsp
- Vanilla extract: a dash
- Salt: a pinch
- Caster sugar: 4 tbsp
- Vegetable oil: 1 tbsp

Directions

1. Put the fruit, lemon juice, and icing sugar in a small cup. Cook for 10 minutes to achieve a saucy texture, then set aside. In a mixing dish, combine the caster sugar, flour, baking powder, and salt.
2. To make a batter, whisk together the almond milk and vanilla extract. Heat 4 teaspoons oil in a nonstick pan and spray it over the entire surface.
3. Add 14 cup of the batter to the pan and cook each side for 3-4 minutes. Serve with a compote.

Traditional Indian Roti

(Ready in 30 minutes | servings 10)

Per serving: Calories; 413; Fat: 26g; Carbs: 38.1g; Protein: 5.6g

Ingredients

- 4 cups bread flour
- 1 teaspoon salt
- 2 teaspoon baking powder
- 3/2 warm water
- 2 cup vegetable oil, for frying

Directions

1. Meticulously combine the flour, baking powder and salt in a mixing bowl. While you thoroughly mix it, add water gradually until the dough stick together
2. Divide the dough into ten balls; create circle with each ball by flattening it.
3. Heat the oil in a frying pan over a flame. Fry the first dough, turn it over while frying, fry until its golden brown.
4. Repeat for the remaining dough.
5. Drain the oil from each Roti by transferring each roti to a paper towel-lined plate to drain the excess oil.

Bon Appetit!

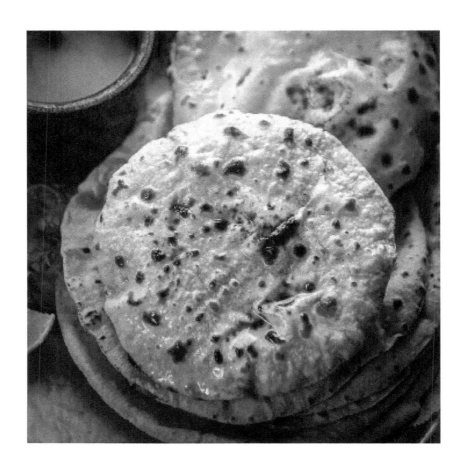

Sweet Coconut Raspberry pancake

Ready in 12 minutes | **Servings:** 4

Ingredients

- 4 tbsp flax seed powder + 12 tbsp water
- 1 cup of coconut milk
- ½ cup fresh raspberries, mashed
- 1 cup oat flour
- 2 tsp baking soda
- A pinch salt
- 2 tbsp coconut sugar
- 4 tbsp pure date syrup
- 1 tsp cinnamon powder
- 4 tbsp unsweetened coconut flakes
- 4 tsp plant butter
- Fresh raspberries for garnishing

Directions

1. Mix the flax seed powder with the water in a medium bowl and thicken for 5 minutes.
2. Mix in the coconut milk and raspberries.
3. Add the oat flour, baking soda, salt, coconut sugar, date syrup, and cinnamon powder. Fold in the coconut flakes until well combined.
4. Working in batches, melt a quarter of the butter in a non-stick skillet and add ¼ cup of the batter. Cook until set beneath and golden brown, 2 minutes.

5. Flip the pancake and cook on the other side until set and golden brown, 2 minutes.
6. Transfer to a plate and make the remaining pancakes using the rest of the ingredients in the same proportions.
7. Garnish the pancakes with some raspberries and serve warm!

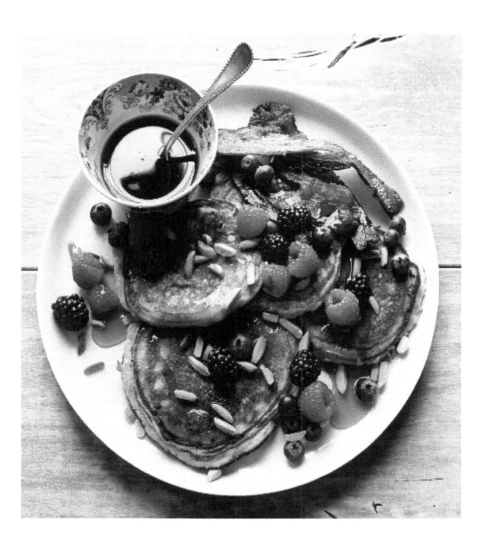

Pineapple French toast

*Preparation Time: **5-15 minutes** | Servings: **8***

Calories 294: Fats 4.7g: Carbs 52.0g: Protein 11.6g

Ingredients
- 4 tbsp flax seed powder + 6 tbsp water
- 3 cups unsweetened almond milk
- 1 cup almond flour
- 4 tbsp pure maple syrup + extra for drizzling
- 4 pinches salt
- 1 tbsp cinnamon powder
- 1 tsp fresh lemon zest
- 2 tbsp fresh pineapple juice
- 16 whole-grain bread slices

Directions
1. Preheat the oven to 400 F and lightly grease a roasting rack with olive oil. Set aside.
2. In a medium bowl, mix the flax seed powder with water and allow thickening for 5 to 10 minutes.
3. Whisk in the almond milk, almond flour, maple syrup, salt, cinnamon powder, lemon zest, and pineapple juice.
4. Soak the bread on both sides in the almond milk mixture and allow sitting on a plate for 2 to 3 minutes.
5. Heat a large skillet over medium heat and place the bread in the pan. Cook until golden brown on the bottom side. Flip the bread and cook further until golden brown on the other side, 4 minutes in total.
6. Transfer to a plate, drizzle some maple syrup on top and serve immediately.

Mushroom Avocado Panini

Preparation Time: 5-15 minutes | Cooking Time: 30 minutes |
Servings: 8
Calories 338. Fats 22. 4g Carbs 25. 5g Protein 12. 4g

Ingredients
- 2 tbsp olive oil
- 2 cup sliced white button mushrooms
- Salt and black pepper to taste
- 2 ripe avocados, pitted, peeled, and sliced
- 4 tbsp freshly squeezed lemon juice
- 2 tbsp chopped parsley
- 1 tsp pure maple syrup
- 16 slices whole-wheat ciabatta
- 8 oz sliced plant-based Parmesan cheese
- 2 tbsp olive oil

Directions
1. Heat the olive oil in a medium skillet over medium heat and sauté the mushrooms until softened, 5 minutes. Season with salt and black pepper. Turn the heat off.
2. Preheat a panini press to medium heat, 3 to 5 minutes.
3. Mash the avocado in a medium bowl and mix in the lemon juice, parsley, and maple syrup.
4. Spread the mixture on 4 bread slices, divide the mushrooms and plant-based Parmesan cheese on top.
5. Cover with the other bread slices and brush the top with olive oil.

6. Grill the sandwiches one after another in the heated press until golden brown and the cheese melted.

Serve warm.

Cheddar Grits with Soy Chorizo

(Ready in 25 minutes / servings 12)

Ingredients

- 2 cup quick-cooking grits
- 1 cup grated plant-based cheddar
- 4 tbsp peanut butter
- 2 cup soy chorizo, chopped
- 2 cup corn kernels
- 4 cups vegetable broth

Directions

1. Oven to be preheated at 380 F.
2. Pour the broth in a pot and bring to a boil over gentle heat. Stir in salt and grits.
3. Lower the heat and cook until the grits are thickened, stirring periodically.
4. Turn the heat off, put in the plant-based cheddar cheese, peanut butter, soy chorizo, corn, and mix well.
5. Spread the mixture into a greased baking dish and bake for 45 minutes until slightly puffed and golden brown. Serve right away.

Enjoy!

CONCLUSION

There is a plethora of compelling reasons to make a positive difference and transition to a plant-based diet. A plant-based diet will increase your quality of life by providing you with more energy and stamina, assisting you in losing excess body weight, and perhaps even extending your time on this magnificent world. Too much energy and fossil fuels are lost in the process of obtaining meat and other animal products, shipping them over miles and miles of road, and refining them. You will also be bringing a genuine and important difference to the future of our planet Earth by making the transition.

By switching to rich plant-based meals, we can save the earth and also take care of ourselves.

Thank you for taking time to read this.

Lightning Source UK Ltd.
Milton Keynes UK
UKHW020655020421
381422UK00001B/11